ESSENTIAL GUIDE TO GRANULOMA ANNULARE

Comprehensive Insights and Practical
Approaches for Patients and
Practitioners

DR. CASEY LOREN

© 2024 by CASEY LOREN

All rights reserved .Except for brief quotations included in critical reviews and certain other noncommercial uses allowed by copyright law, no part of this book may be reproduced, distributed, or transmitted in any form or by any means, including photocopying, recording, or other electronic or mechanical methods, without the publisher's prior written permission.

DISCLAIMER

This book's content is only meant to be used for general informative purposes. Although the author has taken great care to ensure the content is accurate and thorough, no warranties or assurances on the information's accuracy, correctness, or reliability are provided. It is recommended that readers employ their own judgment and discretion when applying any material found in this book to their particular situation.

The information in this book is not intended to replace professional advice, nor is the author an expert in any of the subjects covered. It is recommended that readers consult with experienced professionals regarding any particular issues or concerns.

Any name that may be mentioned or referred in this book does not imply endorsement, recommendation, or relationship on the part of the author with any person, entity, good, website, or association. These references are made only for informational purposes and are not meant to be taken as recommendations or endorsements.

The information contained in this book may cause readers to suffer loss or damage, for which the author disclaims all obligation and accountability. The only people accountable for the decisions and actions taken by readers using the information presented are themselves.

Any names, characters, companies, locations, activities, occasions, and incidents referenced in this book are either made up or the result of the author's imagination. Any likeness to real people, living or dead, or to real things is entirely coincidental.

This book's content may change at any time, without prior notice, according to the author.

The onus is on the reader to verify whether there have been any updates or revisions.

The reader accepts the conditions of this disclaimer by reading this book. Please do not read this book or use its contents if you do not agree to these terms.

Table of Contents

CHAPTER 1 14

   KNOWLEDGE OF GRANULOMA ANNULARE 14

   Reasons and Danger Factors: 15

   Symptoms and Indications: 16

   The following complications are linked to Granuloma Annulare: 17

   Current Studies and Advancements: 18

CHAPTER 2 20

   VARIANTS AND CLINICAL PRESENTATION 20

   Crucial Reference for Granuloma Annulare 20

   Granuloma Annulare Generalised 21

   Clinical Characteristics 22

   Perforating Annulare Granuloma 23

   Granuloma Annulare Subcutaneous 24

   Unusual Forms and Uncommon Variants ...25

   Granuloma Annulare in Paediatrics.............26

Granuloma Annulare in Senior Individuals . 27

Comorbidities and Coexisting Conditions ... 29

Images for Illustrations and Case Studies ... 30

Identifying Trends and Advancement 31

CHAPTER 3 34

IMMUNOLOGY AND PATHOPHYSIOLOGY 34

Essential Guide on Immunology and Pathophysiology of Granuloma Annulare 34

Inflammatory Routes Associated With 36

Immunological Reactions in Granuloma Annulare 37

The Function of Immunity 37

Hereditary Propensities 38

Environmental Stressors 39

Results of Immunohistochemistry 40

Profiles of Cytokines 41

Changes in Vascular Angiogenesis 42

Prospects for Further Pathophysiology Research..................42

CHAPTER 4 46
PROCEDURES FOR DIAGNOSIS 46

Crucial Manual for Granuloma Annulare: Diagnostic Techniques 46

Comprehensive Background....................47

Granuloma Annulare Dermoscopy 48

Skin Biopsy Methodologies 49

Histological Discoveries 50

Lab Examinations and Research 51

Imaging investigations (MRI, ultrasound, X-ray) 52

Diverse Diagnostic Techniques 53

Algorithmic Methodology...................53

Analysing Diagnostic Findings................54

Difficulties with Diagnosis....................55

Multidisciplinary Diagnosis Approach.........56

CHAPTER 5 58

METHODS OF TREATMENT 58

Topical Interventions 58

Injections into the Lesions 60

Oral Medications for Systemic Therapies 60

Options for Phototherapy 62

Surgical Procedures 62

Laser Treatment 63

New Therapeutic Approaches and Biological Agents 64

Complementary Medicines 64

Algorithms and Guidelines for Treatment ... 65

Handling Side Effects of Treatment 65

CHAPTER 6 68

PATIENT INSTRUCTION AND LIFESTYLE GUIDANCE 68

Crucial Reference for Granuloma Annulare 68

Coping Mechanisms for Impact on Emotions 69

Skincare Advice 70

UV Exposure and Sun Protection 71

Nutrition and Dietary Guidelines................. 72

Guidelines for Physical Activity and Exercise 73

Stress Reduction Methods 73

Resources and Support Groups 74

Including Treatment in Everyday Activities. 75

Planning for Long-Term Management......... 76

CHAPTER 7 78

    PEDIATRIC POINTS TO REMEMBER 78

Crucial Manual for Paediatric Granuloma Annulare 78

Diagnostic Difficulties in Kids 79

Paediatric Patient Treatment Methods........ 80

Effect on Children's Quality of Life 81

Long-Term Outlook and Sustaining 82

Care for Paediatric Dermatology.................. 83

Interacting with Parents and Paediatric Patients 84

Family-Friendly Educational Resources......85

Making the Switch to Adult Care 85

Paediatric Dermatology Research and Innovation 86

CHAPTER 8...88

Granelloma Annulare in Senior Individuals 88

Clinical Display...88

Epidemiology..89

Comorbidities and Age-Related Changes 90

Treatment Difficulties for Seniors 91

Options for Treatment 91

Senior Dermatology Services 92

Issues with Life Quality 93

Involvement of Family and Carers...............94

Ethical Issues in Dermatology for the Elderly 94

Research on Geriatric Dermatology's Future Directions..95

CHAPTER 9...98

EFFECTS OF PSYCHOLOGY AND LIFE QUALITY 98

Granuloma Annulare's Psychological Impact 98

Effect on Self-Esteem and Body Image 99

Social Interactions and Relationships 99

Modifications to Career and Lifestyle 100

Obtaining Mental Health Assistance 101

Evaluations of Quality of Life 101

Results as stated by Patients 102

Psychosocial Intervention Research 102

Enhancing Health of Patients 103

CHAPTER 10 106
RESEARCH DEVELOPMENTS AND UPCOMING PATHS 106

Current Research Results 106

Investigations into Granuloma Annulare Genome 107

Discovery of Biomarkers 107

In development are targeted therapies 108

Methods for Patient Stratification..............109

Collaborative Research Projects.................109

Funding for Research and Patient Advocacy 110

Clinical Trials and Ethical Issues.................110

Opportunities for Translational Research...111

Prospects for Granuloma Annulare Management in the Future.........................112

CHAPTER 1
KNOWLEDGE OF GRANULOMA ANNULARE

A very rare chronic skin ailment called Granuloma Annulare (GA) is characterized by the production of small, solid bumps or nodules in the form of rings or arcs on the skin. Although these lesions can form anywhere on the body and range in size, they most frequently affect the hands, feet, elbows, and knees.

Granuloma Annulare Types:

1. The most prevalent kind, known as localized Granuloma Annulare, is distinguished by solitary patches of lesions.

2. Generalised Granuloma Annulare: This kind of affects numerous body parts and causes extensive lesions.

3. Granuloma Annulare subcutaneous: In this variation, the lesions develop beneath the skin as opposed to on the surface.

Reasons and Danger Factors:

Although the precise cause of Granuloma Annulare is unknown, the following factors could be involved:

- Immune responses

- Heredity

- Specific drugs

- Contaminations

- Sun exposure

A family history of the ailment, being female, and having certain underlying medical conditions including diabetes or thyroid issues are risk factors for developing Granuloma Annulare.

Symptoms and Indications:

Raised, reddish-colored, or skin-colored pimples that occur in a ring or circular pattern are the main signs of Granuloma Annulare. Although they are mostly harmless, these lesions sometimes itch. There could be just one lesion in certain situations, or there might be several lesions.

Granuloma Annulare diagnosis:

A dermatologist would usually perform a physical examination of the skin lesions to diagnose Granuloma Annulare. A biopsy may be necessary in some circumstances to confirm the diagnosis. To rule out further potential causes, imaging examinations or blood tests may also be prescribed.

Diagnostic Differentiation:

Other skin disorders like ringworm, erythema multiforme, and sarcoidosis can mimic Granuloma Annulare. Making the distinction between these illnesses requires a comprehensive assessment by a medical expert.

The following complications are linked to Granuloma Annulare:

Granuloma Annulare is usually benign and does not result in life-threatening health issues, but if the lesions are large or prominently displayed, they may cause cosmetic issues as well as other consequences.

Prevalence and Epidemiology:

Granuloma Annulare is regarded as rare, with an incidence in the general population estimated to be 1 in 1,000. Although it can happen at any age, children and young adults are more likely to experience it.

Current Studies and Advancements:

Research on Granuloma Annulare is ongoing with the goal of better understanding the underlying causes of the condition and creating more potent treatments. Research may examine the significance of immunological dysfunction, hereditary variables, and possible targeted treatments.

Overview of Treatment Options:

The kind and intensity of the lesions determine the course of treatment for Granuloma Annulare. Possible choices could be:

- Watching without intervention, since many situations end on their own

- Topical corticosteroids to lessen irritation and inflammation

- Localised lesions treated with intrathecal corticosteroid injections

The use of UV light in phototherapy

- Oral treatments for widespread or resistant instances, such as retinoids or antimalarials

- Laser or cryotherapy treatment for certain lesions

Granuloma Annulare patients must collaborate closely with medical professionals to choose the best course of action for them given their unique circumstances.

CHAPTER 2

VARIANTS AND CLINICAL PRESENTATION

Crucial Reference for Granuloma Annulare

Localized, ring-shaped lesions are the hallmark of the benign, persistent dermatological disorder known as granuloma annulare (GA). The ailment is comparatively infrequent and manifests in multiple unique clinical manifestations. An in-depth description of every GA variation, its clinical manifestation, and related variables is given in this handbook.

Localised Annulare Granuloma

Synopsis

About 75% of GA cases are classified as localized granuloma annulare. This is the most frequent type of the condition. Usually, it appears as one or more clear-centered, ring-shaped plaques.

Clinical Characteristics

- **Lesion Appearance:** Firm, little papules arranged in a ring configuration.

- **Common Places:** The ankles, wrists, hands, and feet.

Age of Onset: Although it can happen at any age, children and young people experience it most frequently.

Identification and Handling

- **Diagnosis:** Skin biopsy and/or clinical examination.

Treatment: Usually self-limiting; therapy may not be necessary. Using topical steroids can help relieve symptoms.

Granuloma Annulare Generalised

Synopsis

Lesions are prevalent in generalized granuloma annulare, which is less common than the localized type.

Clinical Characteristics

Appearance of Lesion: Several tiny, flesh-colored, or erythematous papules that may combine to form bigger plaques.

- **Common Places:** The arms, legs, and trunk.

Age of Onset: Individuals, especially middle-aged and older individuals, are more likely to experience it.

Identification and Handling

Diagnosis: To rule out systemic disorders, a clinical examination, a skin biopsy, and sometimes blood testing are necessary.

Treatment: May be more difficult to manage. Intralesional corticosteroids, oral drugs (such as isotretinoin and antimalarials), and systemic therapies including phototherapy are available options.

Perforating Annulare Granuloma

Synopsis

In a rare variation known as perforating granuloma annulare, collagen tends to be expelled through the epidermis by the lesions.

Clinical Characteristics

- **Appearance of Lesion:** Umbilicated nodules or papules with a crust or scale in the center.

- **Common Locations:** Can occur anywhere on the body, however it usually affects the hands and fingers.

- **Age of Onset:** May have an impact on adults and youngsters alike.

Identification and Handling

- **Diagnosis:** Transepidermal collagen elimination was shown by clinical examination and biopsy.

- **Treatment:** As for other kinds, but with a focus on controlling the risk of subsequent infection because of open lesions.

Granuloma Annulare Subcutaneous

Synopsis

Children are primarily affected with subcutaneous granuloma annulare, also referred to as deep granuloma annulare.

Clinical Characteristics

- **Lesion Appearance:** Subcutaneous tissue contains firm, painless nodules.

- **Common Locations:** Usually found on the scalp, buttocks, and lower extremities.

Age of Onset: Mostly in young people.

Identification and Handling

The diagnosis was made using a biopsy, imaging (MRI or ultrasound), and clinical evaluation.

Adjustment: Frequently self-limiting. For cosmetic or diagnostic purposes, surgical excision may be considered.

Unusual Forms and Uncommon Variants

Synopsis

Rare variations and atypical forms include papular GA, perforating GA, and linear GA.

Clinical Characteristics

- **Lesion Appearance:** May differ greatly; papular GA appears as little papules without a distinct ring, whereas linear GA presents along a dermatome.

Common Locations: Varies according to the particular version.

- **Age of Onset:** All age groups are susceptible.

Identification and Handling

Diagnosis: Necessitates a comprehensive clinical assessment and biopsy.

- **Treatment:** based on the particular form and intensity; may include phototherapy, systemic, or topical interventions.

Granuloma Annulare in Paediatrics

Synopsis

GA is more likely to be localized or subcutaneous in pediatric patients, and it frequently manifests differently in adult cases.

Clinical Characteristics

- **Lesion Appearance:** Usually localized or subcutaneous, but commonly resembling adult presentations.

Common Locations: The scalp, hands, foot, and buttocks.

Age of Onset: Most common in kids between the ages of 2 and 10.

Identification and Handling

* **Diagnosis:** Clinical assessment and biopsy may be necessary.

Adjustment: Frequently self-limiting. Common methods include observation or topical steroids.

Granuloma Annulare in Senior Individuals

Synopsis

In older people, GA may manifest in unusual or generalized forms and may be linked to systemic illnesses.

Clinical Characteristics

Appearance of Lesions: Broad lesions that could be more chronic and widespread.

- **Common Places:** The arms, legs, and trunk.

Age of Onset: Usually more than fifty years old.

Identification and Handling

The clinical examination, biopsy, and search for underlying systemic problems led to the **diagnosis**.

Treatment: Comorbid conditions must be closely monitored; systemic medications are frequently necessary.

Comorbidities and Coexisting Conditions

Synopsis

GA is linked to several systemic illnesses, especially when it comes to unusual or generalized forms.

Typical Connections

Diabetes Mellitus: Particularly in cases of GA.

- **Thyroid Disorder:** In both hyper- and hypothyroid conditions.

- Dyslipidemia: Unusual cholesterol levels.

- **Autoimmune Diseases:** Conditions like systemic lupus erythematosus and rheumatoid arthritis.

Identification and Handling

With a thorough history, physical examination, and pertinent laboratory testing, the **diagnosis** has been made.

- **Treatment:** Managing GA may involve addressing the underlying comorbid condition.

Images for Illustrations and Case Studies

Synopsis

Case studies and visual documentation are essential for comprehending the many ways that GA is presented.

Usability

- **Photographs:** Aid in identifying various GA types and setting them apart from other dermatoses.

- **Case Studies:** Offer information on the course, effects of treatment, and distinct GA manifestations.

References

- **Dermatology Atlases:** Excellent resources for fine-grained case descriptions and excellent photos.

Clinical reviews and case reports are published in **Medical Journals**.

Identifying Trends and Advancement

Synopsis

Diagnosing and treating GA are aided by knowledge of its usual patterns and course.

Important Details

- **First Lesions:** Usually start as little papules.

- **Progression:** Could stay localized or spread to other areas.

Resolution: May clear up on its own or last for years, frequently with intervals of remission and recurrence.

Identification and Handling

Observation: Consistently keeping an eye out for any new or altered symptoms.

Intervention: Modified care according to the degree and influence on the patient's quality of life.

This thorough guide emphasizes the significance of identifying granuloma annulare's numerous forms and related disorders, making it a vital tool for treating the condition and helping professionals and patients understand it.

CHAPTER 3
IMMUNOLOGY AND PATHOPHYSIOLOGY

Essential Guide on Immunology and Pathophysiology of Granuloma Annulare

A benign, long-term dermatological disorder called granuloma annulare (GA) is typified by localized or widespread annular (ring-shaped) plaques or nodules. It is essential to comprehend the immunological and pathophysiological features of GA to diagnose and treat the condition effectively. This guide explores many facets of the immunology and pathophysiology of GA.

Immunological Processes

multinucleated giant cells or epithelioid cells, which are characteristic of granulomatous inflammation.

Inflammatory Routes Associated With

Several important processes are involved in the inflammatory pathways in GA:

1. **NF-κB Pathway**: This transcription factor pathway is essential for the production of genes that promote inflammation and is triggered in response to inflammatory cytokines.

2. **JAK-STAT route**: This route contributes to the activation and growth of immune cells as well as mediating the actions of different cytokines.

3. **MAPK route**: This route plays a role in immunological responses and inflammation by influencing how cells react to growth factors, cytokines, and stress.

The primary cause of granuloma annulare is the intricate interaction of immune systems. Important elements consist of:

1. **T-cell Mediated Response**: T-cells are thought to be involved in the development of GA. T-cells that have been activated, namely CD4+ helper T-cells, penetrate the dermis and are essential for starting and sustaining the inflammatory response.

2. **Cytokine Production**: IFN-γ, TNF-α, and IL-1 are among the cytokines released by activated T-cells. These cytokines attract and activate macrophages and other immune cells, which in turn causes the formation of granulomas.

3. **Macrophage Activation**: Foreign materials and cellular waste are ingested by macrophages, which are then stimulated by cytokines to create the distinctive granulomas of GA. These macrophages can differentiate into

Immunological Reactions in Granuloma Annulare

Numerous cellular reactions are involved in granuloma annulare:

1. **Langerhans Cells**: These epidermal antigen-presenting cells present antigens to T-cells, thereby starting an immunological response.

2. **Keratinocytes**: These skin cells can contribute to the local inflammatory environment by producing chemokines and cytokines.

3. **Fibroblasts**: Activated fibroblasts contribute to tissue remodeling and granuloma development by producing cytokines and extracellular matrix components.

The Function of Immunity

It is believed that autoimmune factors contribute to GA:

1. **Autoantigen Presentation**: An autoimmune reaction may be triggered by antigen-presenting cells' aberrant presentation of self-antigens.

2. **Autoantibodies**: Compared to other autoimmune disorders, GA is less well-characterized when it comes to the potential involvement of autoantibodies that target certain skin components.

3. **Association with Other Autoimmune Conditions**: Patients with thyroiditis and type 1 diabetes have also been seen to have GA, indicating a common autoimmune tendency.

Hereditary Propensities

People may be predisposed to GA by genetic factors:

1. **HLA Associations**: Research has linked specific HLA alleles to an increased risk of GA, indicating a hereditary predisposition to the illness.

2. **Family History**: A genetic predisposition may be indicated if there is a history of GA or other autoimmune illnesses in the family.

3. **Genetic Mutations**: Certain genetic mutations that impact skin integrity and immunological modulation may have a role in the development of GA.

Environmental Stressors

There are environmental factors that might cause or worsen GA.

1. **Infections**: Viral, fungal, or bacterial infections can replicate a trigger's molecular structure or stimulate the immune system.

2. **Drugs**: The start of GA has been associated with some drugs, including TNF-α inhibitors and allopurinol.

3. **Stress**: Insect bites and tattoos are examples of physical stress to the skin that can result in the formation of GA lesions.

Results of Immunohistochemistry

The results of immunohistochemical examination of GA lesions are as follows:

1. **Cellular Markers**: T-cells and macrophages within the lesions can be identified by immunostaining for CD3, CD4, CD8, and CD68.

2. **Cytokine Expression**: The presence of cytokines such as TNF-α, IL-1, and IFN-γ in the inflammatory milieu can be shown by immunohistochemical staining.

3. **Matrix Components**: The alterations in the dermal structure linked to GA can be emphasized by staining for collagen and other extracellular matrix elements.

Profiles of Cytokines

In GA, cytokine profiles are typified by:

1. **Pro-inflammatory Cytokines**: TNF-α, IL-1, and IFN-γ are frequently detected at elevated levels in GA lesions, which promote inflammation.

2. **Anti-inflammatory Cytokines**: The body may produce cytokines that reflect its efforts to control and alleviate inflammation, such as IL-10.

3. **Chemokines**: Chemokines that induce inflammation, such as CXCL9 and CXCL10, draw immune cells to the location and aid in the granulomatous reaction.

Changes in Vascular Angiogenesis

The vasculature changes in GA lesions:

1. **Increased Vascularization**: GA lesions frequently exhibit an increase in blood vessel development, which facilitates the infiltration of immune cells.

2. **Endothelial Cell Activation**: Leukocyte migration into the skin is aided by the expression of adhesion molecules by activated endothelial cells.

3. **Vascular Permeability**: Immune cells and plasma proteins can permeate into the afflicted tissue due to increased blood vessel permeability.

Prospects for Further Pathophysiology Research

Prospective avenues for investigating the pathogenesis of GA encompass:

1. **Genomic Studies**: By identifying genetic variants and mutations linked to GA, cutting-edge genomic tools can shed light on the disease's inherited characteristics.

2. **Molecular Pathways**: New treatment targets may be found by examining the molecular pathways connected to the production of granulomas.

3. **Immunomodulatory Therapies**: By focusing on modifying particular elements of the immune response, targeted immunotherapies may be developed that provide better outcomes with fewer adverse effects.

4. **Biomarkers**: Personalised treatment approaches and illness monitoring can be enhanced by identifying biomarkers for disease activity and response to therapy.

5. **Microbiota Studies**: Investigating how the skin and gut microbiota function in GA may help identify new pathogenic pathways and treatment targets.

It is essential to comprehend the complex immunological and pathophysiological features of granuloma annulare to create more efficient diagnostic methods and therapeutic interventions. Future patient outcomes may be improved as a result of the intricacies of this disorder being explored by ongoing studies.

CHAPTER 4

PROCEDURES FOR DIAGNOSIS

Crucial Manual for Granuloma Annulare: Diagnostic Techniques

The benign, long-term dermatological disorder known as Granuloma Annulare (GA) is characterized by annular (ring-shaped) plaques or nodules on the skin. To differentiate GA from other skin disorders and to ensure appropriate care, an accurate diagnosis is essential. Here, we offer a comprehensive guide to the GA diagnostic processes.

Methods of Physical Examination

Visual Examining

- **Lesion Characteristics**: Mostly on the hands, feet, elbows, and knees, look for ring-shaped, skin-colored to erythematous plaques or nodules.

- **Distribution**: Take note of the usual sites (dorsal hands and feet) as well as any unusual sites that could point to distinct types of GA (generalized, subcutaneous, perforating).

Feeling

- **Texture and Consistency**: Evaluate the lesions' firmness, as they might range from soft nodules to firm ones.

- **Tenderness**: Look for any tenderness, as GA tends to lack it.

Comprehensive Background

- **Onset and Duration**: Keep track of the lesions' beginning and length.

- **Symptoms**: Ask about any pain or itching (which are typically absent in GA).

- **Previous Treatments**: Examine any prior medical interventions and their results.

Granuloma Annulare Dermoscopy

Features of the Dermis

- **Colour Patterns**: The granulomas are represented by patches that are yellowish, brownish, or white.

- **Vascular Patterns**: Determine whether a vessel is linear or dotted.

- **Edge Features**: Look for a distinct border, frequently featuring a central clearing.

Diagnostic Worth

Accuracy: Dermoscopy aids in distinguishing GA from other comparable ailments, such as psoriasis and tinea corporis.

- **Non-Invasive**: This technique offers a non-invasive way to support diagnosis.

Skin Biopsy Methodologies

Indications

Atypical Presentations: If the patient presents unusually or if conventional treatments are not working, then a biopsy should be performed.

Histological Confirmation: Required to make a conclusive diagnosis.

Methods

Punch Biopsy: Usually 3–4 mm in diameter, encompassing both healthy and diseased skin.

- **Excisional Biopsy**: To properly evaluate larger lesions, an excisional biopsy may be necessary.

Method

- **Set Up**: Cleanse and numb the skin.

- **Biopsy**: Remove a core of tissue with a punch tool.

- **Closure**: Depending on the size, suture or let to heal by secondary aim.

Histological Discoveries

Granulomas

- **Pattern**: Palisading granulomas accompanied by core necrobiosis, or collagen degradation.

- **Cell Types**: Lymphocytes surrounding necrobiotic foci, multinucleated giant cells, and histocytes.

Discoloration

- **Hematoxylin and Eosin (H&E)**: Illustrates the distinctive histological characteristics.

On rare occasions, **Special Stains** are required to rule out infections or other diseases.

Lab Examinations and Research

Regular Blood Testing

Complete Blood Count (CBC): Generally normal, but useful in ruling out illnesses of the system.

- **Erythrocyte Sedimentation Rate (ESR)**: Increased in circumstances involving systemic inflammation.

Particular Examinations

Given the correlation between GA and diabetes, especially in widespread cases, **Diabetes Screening** is recommended.

- **Autoimmune Panels**: To exclude rheumatoid arthritis and lupus among other illnesses.

Imaging investigations (MRI, ultrasound, X-ray)

X-Ray

Indications: Infrequently used but beneficial when bone involvement is present (subcutaneous GA).

Results: Generally normal; soft tissue nodules may be visible.

MRI

- **Indications**: thorough examination of deep lesions or if alternative diagnoses are taken into account.

- **Results**: On T1-weighted images, a soft tissue mass with low to intermediate signal strength.

Ultrasound

- **Indications**: Assessment of nodules beneath the skin.

Results: The granulomas correspond to hypoechoic or anechoic locations.

Diverse Diagnostic Techniques

Typical Disparities

- **Tinea Corporis**: Fungal infection characterized by ring-shaped lesions, frequently accompanied by center clearing and scaling.

- **Psoriasis**: Widespread, frequently more symmetrical erythematous plaques with silvery scales.

- **Sarcoidosis**: Granulomatous illness that typically involves systemic circulation and can resemble GA.

Algorithmic Methodology

1. **History and Physical Examination**: First evaluation to pinpoint distinguishing characteristics.

2. **Dendroscopy**: To fine-tune the diagnosis.

3. **Biopsy**: If necessary, for histological confirmation.

4. **Laboratory Tests**: To rule out conditions related to the system.

5. **Imaging**: For unusual or deeply situated lesions.

Analysing Diagnostic Findings

Histopathology

The diagnosis of palisading granulomas with central necrobiosis is **positive diagnosis**.

Uncertain or Negative Outcomes: May call for a second biopsy or different diagnostic modalities.

Lab Examinations

Normal Results: Common in GA that is localized.

Anomalous Outcomes: This could point to a systemic illness that needs more research.

Visual Aids

Normal Findings: In localized GA, expected.

- **Abnormal Findings**: Indicate a more thorough involvement or a different diagnosis.

Difficulties with Diagnosis

Unusual Demonstrations

GA may exhibit - **Variable Morphology**: unusual forms, sizes, and locations.

- **Overlap with Other Conditions**: This condition resembles other dermatological conditions in appearance.

Variability in Histology

Lesions that are treated or that were discovered early may exhibit non-specific inflammatory alterations.

- **Sampling Errors**: An incorrect diagnosis may result from insufficient biopsy samples.

Multidisciplinary Diagnosis Approach

Cooperation

Dermatologists: Play a major part in both diagnosis and treatment.

Pathologists: Essential for confirmation of histopathology.

Endocrinologists: For the treatment of related illnesses such as diabetes.

- **Rheumatologists**: When there is a possibility of autoimmune connections.

Coordinated Healthcare

Case Conferences: Consistent gatherings to deliberate on complex cases.

- **Shared Records**: Ensuring that patient data is accessible to all members of the team to provide coordinated treatment.

A comprehensive clinical examination, in conjunction with dermoscopy, biopsy, and relevant laboratory and imaging testing, is necessary for the diagnosis of Granuloma Annulare. For an accurate diagnosis and successful treatment, a systematic and multidisciplinary approach is necessary due to the condition's varied presentation and overlap with other disorders.

CHAPTER 5
METHODS OF TREATMENT

The benign, frequently self-limiting dermatological disorder known as Granuloma Annulare (GA) is characterized by reddish, ring-shaped skin pimples. Although the precise etiology is still unknown, immunological response is thought to be involved. To ensure a clear and competent knowledge, this book offers a thorough overview of the various treatment options for GA.

Topical Interventions

1. **Anabolic Agents**:

- **Mechanism**: In the afflicted skin area, topical corticosteroids function by lowering inflammation and inhibiting the immunological response.

Usage: Usually used as ointments or creams. For lesions that are bigger or more extensive, doctors may give strong steroids.

- **Common Steroids**: betamethasone, clobetasol, and hydrocortisone.

- **Side Effects**: Hypopigmentation, stretch marks (striae), skin thinning (atrophy), and elevated risk of skin infections.

2. **Inhibitors of Calcineurin**:

Mechanism: By inhibiting calcineurin, these drugs lessen the activation of T cells and the release of cytokines, which in turn reduces inflammation.

Usage: Appropriate for delicate regions such as the face or intertriginous zones where the use of steroids may result in notable adverse reactions.

- **Common Inhibitors** : Pimecrolimus (Elidel), Tacrolimus (Protopic).

Side Effects: Rare cases of cancer with prolonged use, burning sensation, and itching at the application site.

Injections into the Lesions

- **Method**: Involves injecting corticosteroids straight into the lesions caused by granuloma annulare.

- Triamcinolone acetonide is a common agent.

Benefits: quicker reaction time, increased local concentration, direct administration to the lesion.

- **Side Effects**: White spots (hypopigmentation), localized skin atrophy, and pain at the injection site.

Oral Medications for Systemic Therapies

1. **Adrenoceptors**:

- **Indication**: For GA that is widespread or progressing quickly.

- Prednisone is a common agent.

Side Effects: mood swings, weight gain, osteoporosis, hypertension, and hyperglycemia.

2. **Antimalarials**:

Mechanism: Said to control the immune response and lessen inflammatory responses.

Common Agents: Chloroquine and hydroxychloroquine.

- **Side Effects**: Skin rash, gastrointestinal issues, and retinal toxicity (needs routine eye checks).

3. **Antibiotics**:

Mechanism: Antibacterial and anti-inflammatory qualities combined.

- **Common Agents**: minocycline and dapsone.

- **Side Effects**: Photosensitivity, gastrointestinal problems, hemolysis in G6PD deficiency (dapsone).

Options for Phototherapy

- **Types**: Psoralen in combination with UVA (PUVA), Ultraviolet B (UVB), and Ultraviolet A (UVA).

- **Mechanism**: Through carefully monitored UV light exposure, modifies immune response and lowers inflammation.

- **Usage**: Usually given multiple times a week in a therapeutic environment.

- **Side Effects**: Dryness, erythema, aging of the skin, and an increased risk of skin cancer with continued use.

Surgical Procedures

Indication: When there are serious concerns about appearance or for lesions that are resistant.

- **Procedures**: curettage and excision.

- **Benefits**: Lesions are immediately removed.

- **Side Effects**: Infection, scarring, and chance of recurrence.

Laser Treatment

- **Types**: CO_2 laser, pulsed dye laser.

- **Mechanism**: Causes localized granulomatous tissue damage by targeting particular chromophores in the skin.

- **Benefits**: accuracy and low invasiveness.

- **Side Effects**: Risk of pigmentation changes, edema, and redness.

New Therapeutic Approaches and Biological Agents

- **Biologics**: Target certain immune system components; examples include interleukin inhibitors (like ustekinumab) and TNF-alpha inhibitors (like adalimumab).

- **Advantages**: Targeted method of treatment, may be helpful for refractory situations.

- **Difficulties**: Expensive, uncertain long-term safety, risk of dangerous infections.

Complementary Medicines

- **Approach**: Combining various therapeutic techniques to increase effectiveness and lessen adverse effects.

- **Instances**: Systemic corticosteroids combined with phototherapy, topical steroids combined with calcineurin inhibitors.

- **Advantages**: Combined effects, and individualized treatment regimens for each patient's need.

Algorithms and Guidelines for Treatment

- **First Assessment**: Determine the scope, location, and effects of GA on the individual.

- **First-Line Treatments**: For localized disease, topical steroids or calcineurin inhibitors.

- **Second-Line Treatments**: Systemic medicines or intralesional injections for particularly severe or resistant situations.

Special Considerations: Age of the patient, co-occurring conditions, adverse effects of treatment, and patient preference.

Handling Side Effects of Treatment

Monitoring: Follow-up appointments regularly to check for adverse effects, especially in the case of systemic therapy.

Preventive Measures - Regular eye checkups for antimalarial users and use of sun protection during phototherapy.

- **Patient Education**: Educating patients about possible adverse effects and warning indications of problems.

Symptom Management: Treating adverse effects as soon as possible; for example, applying emollients to dryness or analgesics to discomfort at the injection site.

Healthcare professionals can effectively manage granuloma annulare by customizing interventions to meet the needs of each patient and maximizing results by being aware of various treatment options.

CHAPTER 6

PATIENT INSTRUCTION AND LIFESTYLE GUIDANCE

Crucial Reference for Granuloma Annulare

Informing Patients about Annulare Granuloma

A benign, long-term skin ailment called Granuloma Annulare (GA) is typified by ring-shaped, reddish-purple pimples or patches on the skin. Though it can happen anywhere on the body, it usually affects the hands, feet, elbows, or knees. Although the precise origin of GA is uncertain, immune system activation is believed to be a contributing factor. GA is not contagious, typically resolves on its own without therapy, and is not linked to other health issues.

Coping Mechanisms for Impact on Emotions

Having a noticeable skin condition such as GA can make daily life emotionally taxing. It's possible for patients to feel embarrassed, self-conscious, or frustrated. Here are a few coping mechanisms:

- **Education**: Patients who are aware of the disease are better able to control their anxiety.

- **Support Networks**: Talking with loved ones, close friends, or support groups can offer consolation on an emotional level as well as useful guidance.

- **Counselling**: In addition to addressing related mental health concerns, professional treatment can assist patients in creating coping strategies.

Mindfulness and Relaxation Techniques: Deep breathing exercises, yoga, meditation, and other similar practices can help lower stress and enhance emotional health.

Skincare Advice

To manage GA, proper skin care is essential:

- **Repeat Moisturising**: Hydrating the skin can lessen irritation and enhance its appearance.

- **Gentle Cleaning**: To prevent additional irritation, use gentle soaps without smell.

Avoid Scratching: Scratching can make the illness worse and result in further infections. If you find yourself scratching as you sleep, keep your nails clipped and think about wearing gloves at night.

- **Topical Treatments**: If your doctor prescribes any topical treatment, such as corticosteroids or other lotions, heed their advice.

UV Exposure and Sun Protection

Everyone should use sun protection, but people with skin disorders should specifically do so:

Sunscreen: Make sure you're wearing a broad-spectrum sunscreen with at least 30 SPF. Every two hours, or more frequently if you're sweating or swimming, reapply.

- **Protective Clothing**: To protect your skin from harsh sunlight, put on long sleeves, caps, and sunglasses.

- **Shade**: Look for cover from the sun throughout the hottest parts of the day, which are usually starting at 10 a.m. until 4 p.m.

- **Avoid Tanning Beds**: These raise the risk of skin cancer and aggravate existing skin disorders.

Nutrition and Dietary Guidelines

Although there isn't a diet that can treat GA specifically, a good diet promotes general skin health:

- **Well-Rounded Diet**: Consume a range of entire grains, fruits, vegetables, lean meats, and healthy fats.

Anti-Inflammatory Foods: Flaxseeds, walnuts, salmon, and other foods high in omega-3 fatty acids may all help lower inflammation.

- **Hydration**: To keep your skin moisturized, sip on lots of water.

Reduce Sugar and Processed Foods: These can aggravate skin conditions and lead to inflammation.

Guidelines for Physical Activity and Exercise

Frequent exercise can help with skin conditions and enhance general health:

Stability: Try to get in at least 150 minutes a week of moderate-to-intense or 75 minutes a week of high-intensity exercise.

Exercises with a combination of cardiovascular, strength, and flexibility training should be included.

- **Skin Care During Exercise**: To avoid dry skin, wear clothes that wick away moisture, take a quick shower after working out, and use moisturizer.

Stress Reduction Methods

Stress can make skin disorders like GA worse. Among the things that constitute effective stress management are:

- **Mindfulness & Meditation**: Consistent practice can lower stress and enhance mental well-being.

- **Physical Activity**: Engaging in physical activity helps reduce stress.

- **Hobbies and Leisure Activities**: Indulging in pleasurable pursuits can ease stress and offer a mental respite.

- **Professional Help**: If stress becomes too much to handle, seek advice from mental health specialists.

Resources and Support Groups

Making connections with people who have gone through similar things can be quite helpful:

- **Online Communities**: Social media groups and forums can offer guidance and assistance.

- **Local Support Groups**: To find out about in-person support groups, contact your local hospital or healthcare provider.

Patient Advocacy Organisations: The American Academy of Dermatology and the National Eczema Association are two examples of organizations that can provide information and assistance.

Including Treatment in Everyday Activities

The secret to managing GA is consistency:

- **Routine**: To guarantee adherence, incorporate recommended treatments into your everyday schedule.

Tracking: Record your symptoms, medications, and triggers in a journal to share with your doctor.

- **Communication**: Stay in constant contact with your medical team so that therapies can be modified as necessary.

Planning for Long-Term Management

Proactive management is necessary for long-term success.

Regular Check-ups: To keep an eye on your condition, make regular appointments with your dermatologist.

Adaptability: Be ready to modify your treatment strategy in response to treatments and light of your symptoms as necessary.

- **Self-Education**: Remain up to date on any new GA therapies or research.

- **Healthy Lifestyle**: Keep up a nutritious diet, get regular exercise, learn to manage stress, and wear sunscreen.

Patients can effectively control their GA and retain a great quality of life by learning these tactics and applying them to their daily lives.

CHAPTER 7

PEDIATRIC POINTS TO REMEMBER

Crucial Manual for Paediatric Granuloma Annulare

Patterns of Paediatric Granuloma Annulare

The benign inflammatory skin disorder known as granuloma annulare (GA) is characterized by reddish-colored, ring-shaped pimples. GA can manifest in a variety of ways in pediatric patients:

1. **Localised GA**: The most prevalent type, usually affecting the ankles, wrists, hands, and feet dorsally. Plaques that are round or semicircular are lesions.

2. **Generalised GA**: This variant, which is less common in children, entails extensive

lesions over several body areas. Larger plaques may grow from the lesions coming together.

3. **Subcutaneous GA**: Usually affecting youngsters, this type of GA is characterized by firm, painless nodules under the skin, frequently on the scalp or lower limbs.

4. **Perforating GA**: Infrequent in infants, this pattern consists of papules that may exude necrotic material from a central umbilication.

5. **Patch GA**: This variation appears as slightly raised, erythematous patches that are occasionally misdiagnosed as other dermatological disorders.

Diagnostic Difficulties in Kids

Given its varied appearances and similarities to other dermatologic disorders including tinea, eczema, or psoriasis, diagnosing GA in pediatric patients can be difficult. Important diagnostic actions consist of:

1. **Clinical Examination**: A comprehensive assessment of the skin to determine defining characteristics and the spread of lesions.

2. **Histopathology**: Palisading granulomas with core mucin deposition is shown by a skin biopsy, which is indicative of GA.

3. **Differential Diagnosis**: Leaving out other illnesses such as autoimmune diseases (such as lupus), fungal infections, infections, and other granulomatous disorders.

4. **Laboratory Tests**: It may occasionally be necessary to perform tests like KOH prep, fungal cultures, or blood tests to check for systemic involvement.

Paediatric Patient Treatment Methods

The goals of managing GA in children are to reduce symptoms and enhance the appearance of the condition. Options for treatment consist of:

1. **Topical Therapies**: Corticosteroids, tacrolimus, or imiquimod creams are first-line treatments that decrease inflammation and encourage lesion resolution.

2. **Intralesional Injections**: Localised GA may benefit from corticosteroid injections.

3. **Systemic Therapies**: Saved for situations that are severe or extensive. Oral corticosteroids, retinoids, and antimalarials (hydroxychloroquine) are among the options.

4. **Phototherapy**: For generalized GA, narrowband UVB or PUVA therapy may be helpful.

5. **Observation**: Since GA is a benign condition, some cases could end on their own without any help.

Effect on Children's Quality of Life

The following factors may impact children's quality of life due to GA:

1. **Psychosocial Impact**: Being aware of one's skin lesions might cause emotional anguish, social disengagement, and self-consciousness.

2. **Physical Discomfort**: Daily activities may be impeded by lesions causing itching or pain.

3. **Family Dynamics**: Long-term dermatological disorders can strain relationships within the family and require regular trips to the doctor.

Long-Term Outlook and Sustaining

Children with GA typically have a good prognosis; many cases go away on their own in a matter of years. Long-term factors consist of:

1. **Recurrence**: A small percentage of children may need sporadic therapy due to recurrences.

2. **Chronicity**: In rare cases, GA may continue into adulthood and require ongoing care.

3. **Follow-up**: Frequent follow-up appointments to track the development of lesions, how well treatments are working, and any possible adverse drug reactions.

Care for Paediatric Dermatology

For pediatric GA, a multidisciplinary approach is necessary for optimal care:

1. **Paediatric Dermatologists**: Professionals skilled in treating skin disorders in youngsters.

2. **Primary Care Physicians**: Coordinating general health management with primary care.

3. For instruction and supportive treatment, **Allied Health Professionals** include therapists and nurses.

Interacting with Parents and Paediatric Patients

To effectively manage pediatric GA, communication is essential:

1. **Age-appropriate Explanations**: To improve comprehension and cooperation, adjust explanations to the child's developmental stage.

2. **Parental Involvement**: Including parents in decisions about their care, assuring them, and attending to their worries.

3. **Visual Aids**: Illustrating the ailment and the steps involved in treatment with models or photos.

Family-Friendly Educational Resources

Providing learning materials aids in the management of GA in families:

1. **Printed Materials**: Informational pamphlets and brochures describing GA, available treatments, and suggestions for at-home care.

2. **Online Resources**: Trusted websites, videos, and support groups for up-to-date knowledge and neighbourhood assistance.

3. **Workshops and Support Groups**: Creating a network of families dealing with comparable issues.

Making the Switch to Adult Care

Transitioning to adult dermatologic care is crucial for pediatric GA patients:

1. **Transition Planning**: Start conversations to get ready for the change during adolescence.

2. **Coordination of Care**: Making sure adult and pediatric dermatologists continue to treat patients together.

3. **Empowering Patients**: Offering resources for autonomous healthcare navigation and promoting self-management abilities.

Paediatric Dermatology Research and Innovation

Continued investigation and creativity are essential to improving GA treatment:

1. **Clinical Trials**: Taking part in studies looking into novel therapies for GA in children.

2. **Biomarker Studies**: Finding biomarkers to forecast the course of a disease and how well a treatment will work.

3. **Emerging therapy**: Research cutting-edge therapy for refractory situations, such as targeted medicines and biologics.

4. **Collaborative Research**: Registries and multicenter studies to collect extensive data on GA in children.

Through a full grasp of these characteristics, healthcare personnel can effectively address the medical, emotional, and social requirements of pediatric patients with GA, providing comprehensive care.

CHAPTER 8

Granelloma Annulare in Senior Individuals

The benign, long-lasting dermatological disease known as granuloma annulare (GA) is characterized by annular (ring-shaped) plaques with a raised border and central clearance. Even though it can impact people of any age, senior patients may require special considerations in terms of presentation and care. GA may have unusual characteristics and a wider distribution in the elderly population, possibly resembling other dermatological disorders.

Clinical Display

GA can manifest in older people as:

- **Localised GA**: This is the most prevalent type, usually presenting with one or more annular plaques on the knees, elbows, hands, or feet.

- **Generalised GA**: More prevalent in the elderly, this condition is marked by many lesions that can cover a significant portion of the body.

- **Subcutaneous GA**: Firm nodules beneath the skin; uncommon in the elderly.

- **Perforating GA**: Rare, causes umbilicated papules due to transepidermal removal of necrobiotic material.

Epidemiology

GA is more common as people age. This may be brought on by alterations in skin structure, aging-related immune system deterioration, or a rise in comorbid conditions that may put older adults at risk for GA.

Diagnostic Issues in the Elderly Population

When determining a patient's age, GA involves:

Clinical Examination: Characterising lesions of interest.

- **Histopathology**: Necrobiotic granulomas with mucus deposition were discovered through skin biopsy.

- **Differential Diagnosis**: Disqualify diseases like sarcoidosis, rheumatoid nodules, tinea corporis, and necrobiosis lipoidica.

Comorbidities and Age-Related Changes

Age-related skin changes and several comorbidities are common in elderly people, and these factors can affect how GA presents and is managed:

- **Skin Changes**: GA presentation may be impacted by decreased collagen, thinning of the epidermis, and immune system suppression.

- **Comorbidities**: More common in the elderly, conditions like diabetes mellitus, thyroid disorders, and cancers have been linked to GA.

Treatment Difficulties for Seniors

Treating GA in older people can be difficult because:

Medication Tolerability: There is a greater chance of side effects and heightened sensitivity to drugs in older persons.

- **Polypharmacy**: Drug interactions with other drugs taken for co-occurring disorders.

Response to Treatment: Older Patients may react to standard therapies less quickly or strongly.

Options for Treatment

- **Topical Therapies**: calcineurin inhibitors, corticosteroids.

Intralesional Steroids: Beneficial for GA that is localized.

- **Systemic Treatments**: biologics, retinoids, dapsone, or antimalarial medications for refractory or generalized GA.

Phototherapy - Photovoltaic or UVB therapy.

Senior Dermatology Services

Giving dermatological treatment to senior citizens calls for an all-encompassing strategy:

- **Comprehensive Assessment**: Assessing comorbidities, present medications, and general health.

- **Multidisciplinary Approach**: Working together with endocrinologists, primary care doctors, and other experts.

Teaching patients about their ailments, available treatments, and anticipated results is known as **Patient Education**.

Issues with Life Quality

GA can have a major negative influence on an older patient's quality of life, especially if it is widespread or persistent:

- **Physical Discomfort**: Pain, discomfort, or itching due to lesions.

Psychosocial Impact: Visible skin changes cause social isolation, anxiety, and depression.

- **Functional Impairment**: Hand or foot lesions may interfere with day-to-day activities.

Palliative care and supportive measures

To manage GA in older individuals, supportive treatment is crucial, with an emphasis on:

- **Symptom Relief**: Applying pain relief techniques, emollients, and antihistamines to itch.

Psychological Support: To address emotional and psychological issues, consider counseling or joining a support group.

- **Holistic Care**: Meeting needs for social support, mobility, and nutrition.

Involvement of Family and Carers

Effective management of GA in older individuals requires the involvement of family and carers.

- **Education and Training**: Instruction on how to help with everyday care, the condition, and the treatment plan for carers.

Emotional Support: Assisting carers who might be impacted by the patient's illness as well.

- **Coordination of Care**: Making sure that to provide coordinated care, carers are a member of the healthcare team.

Ethical Issues in Dermatology for the Elderly

When treating elderly GA patients, the following ethical concerns arise:

Making sure patients or their proxies are aware of the possible hazards and treatment choices is known as **Informed Consent**.

- **Autonomy**: Taking into account the patient's preferences and wishes while creating a care plan.

- **Beneficence and Non-maleficence**: weighing the possible benefits of treatment against its potential drawbacks, particularly in a vulnerable population.

Justice: Guaranteeing all senior patients fair access to resources and care.

Research on Geriatric Dermatology's Future Directions

To improve care, research in geriatric dermatology is essential, especially for disorders such as GA:

- **Epidemiological Studies**: Gaining knowledge about the risk factors and prevalence of GA in the elderly.

Therapeutic Trials: Assessing the safety and effectiveness of new and current treatments, particularly for the elderly population.

- **Quality of Life Studies**: Evaluating how GA affects people's quality of life and how well interventions to enhance it work.

- **Multidisciplinary Research**: Examining how comorbidities, dermatological disorders, and general health in older adults interact.

Healthcare professionals can improve the understanding, diagnosis, and management of GA in senior patients by concentrating on these areas, which will ultimately improve the patient's quality of life and treatment results.

CHAPTER 9
EFFECTS OF PSYCHOLOGY AND LIFE QUALITY

Granuloma Annulare's Psychological Impact

Granuloma annular (GA) may affect a person's everyday life and appearance, which may have psychological impacts on some. Some patients may experience sadness, anxiety, or depression due to the presence of skin lesions, particularly in visible places. Depending on the intensity of GA, coping mechanisms used by the individual, and co-occurring mental health issues, these psychological impacts can differ significantly.

Patient Coping Strategies

Individuals suffering from GA frequently create coping strategies to handle the psychological effects of their illness. These could be asking for help from friends and family, participating in activities that improve wellbeing and self-esteem, joining support groups or online communities, and practicing mindfulness or relaxation techniques.

Effect on Self-Esteem and Body Image

GA lesions are visible, which may have an impact on one's self-esteem and body image. Some people may experience difficulties in social settings or engage in avoidance behaviors as a result of feeling self-conscious or ashamed about the way their skin looks. Self-help techniques, counseling, or therapy can help treat body image problems associated with GA.

Social Interactions and Relationships

GA can have an impact on social interactions and relationships, especially if people feel stigmatized or have bad feelings about their skin condition. Any negative effects on relationships and social interactions can be lessened by having open communication with loved ones, educating others about GA, and cultivating supportive relationships.

Modifications to Career and Lifestyle

Certain GA patients may need to make changes to their lifestyle or profession, particularly if their lesions are uncomfortable or interfere with their everyday activities. Workplace accommodations, such as flexible scheduling or redesigned duties, can help people with GA continue in their careers. Dietary modifications or stress-reduction strategies can also be included in lifestyle improvements to enhance general well-being.

Obtaining Mental Health Assistance

It is essential for people with GA who are experiencing psychological discomfort to have access to mental health support. This assistance could take the form of psychodermatology-specialized dermatologist consultations, counseling, therapy, or psychiatric treatment. For thorough GA management, it is imperative to guarantee mental health services are both accessible and reasonably priced.

Evaluations of Quality of Life

Assessments of quality of life are useful instruments for determining how GA affects patients' general well-being. These evaluations take into account the functional, social, emotional, and physical facets of life that are impacted by GA. Quality-of-life assessments are used by healthcare professionals to customize treatment programs and patient support initiatives.

Results as stated by Patients

PROs, or patient-reported outcomes, include information about the symptoms, feelings, and results of therapy of patients. Healthcare professionals can better understand the special difficulties faced by GA patients and pinpoint opportunities for improvement in support services and care delivery by gathering PRO data.

Psychosocial Intervention Research

The goal of ongoing research on psychosocial therapies for GA is to improve treatment outcomes and patient well-being. Cognitive-behavioral therapy, mindfulness-based techniques, peer support groups, and instructional materials with an emphasis on self-management and coping mechanisms are a few examples of these approaches.

Enhancing Health of Patients

A multidisciplinary strategy that incorporates psychosocial support, lifestyle modifications, and medical therapies is necessary to improve patient well-being. Enhancing care and improving the general quality of life for people with GA requires cooperation between dermatologists, mental health providers, support groups, and patients.

Healthcare providers and support networks can greatly improve the holistic care and experience of people living with Granuloma Annulare by addressing the psychological impact of GA, putting effective coping strategies into practice, encouraging positive body image and self-esteem, supporting relationships and social interactions, facilitating career and lifestyle adjustments, ensuring access to mental health support, conducting quality of life assessments, leveraging patient-reported outcomes, r

CHAPTER 10
RESEARCH DEVELOPMENTS AND UPCOMING PATHS

Current Research Results

New research on granuloma annulare has illuminated its pathophysiology and possible targets for treatment. Scholars have investigated the part immunological dysregulation plays in the development of GA, especially T-cell-mediated responses. Furthermore, research has indicated that cytokines and chemokines may have a role in the inflammatory process within GA lesions. Innovative imaging modalities have also been used to help diagnose GA and gain a better understanding of its morphological characteristics, such as optical coherence tomography and high-resolution ultrasound.

Investigations into Granuloma Annulare Genome

Genetic insights into the etiology of granuloma annulare have been obtained through genomic investigations. Genetic variations linked to GA vulnerability have been found through the use of genome-wide association studies (GWAS). The intricate interaction between genetic predisposition and environmental factors in GA development has been better-understood thanks to these investigations. In addition, current studies are concentrating on epigenetic changes and how these affect GA pathogenesis.

Discovery of Biomarkers

The goal of biomarker discovery initiatives is to find trustworthy biomarkers for GA diagnosis, prognosis, and evaluation of therapy response. Cytokine profiles, autoantibodies, and genetic markers are examples of potential biomarkers. The identification of new biomarkers of diagnostic and prognostic value in GA is being made easier by developments in omics technologies, such as proteomics and metabolomics.

In development are targeted therapies

Understanding the biology of GA better underpins the development of novel targeted therapeutics. The goal of these treatments is to modify particular molecular targets that are part of the inflammatory cascade observed in GA. Targeted cytokine inhibitors, immunological checkpoint inhibitors, and immunomodulatory drugs are a few examples. To assess the effectiveness and safety of these targeted treatments in GA patients, clinical trials are now being conducted.

Methods for Patient Stratification

Strategies for patient classification are changing to customize GA care. This involves classifying different GA subtypes according to their molecular, histological, and clinical traits. By matching patients with the most relevant therapies, stratification helps customize treatment plans, maximize results, and reduce side effects.

Collaborative Research Projects

Multidisciplinary activities involving clinicians, researchers, patient advocacy groups, and industry partners are part of collaborative research programs. These partnerships encourage the exchange of data, the standardization of research techniques, and the creation of accepted standards for the diagnosis and treatment of GA. Collaborative networks expedite translational research and help recruit participants for clinical trials.

Funding for Research and Patient Advocacy

To help patients and carers, advocate for funds for research, and increase public knowledge of GA, patient advocacy groups are essential. Large-scale clinical trials, biomarker discovery, and the investigation of new therapeutic paths are made possible by increased financing for research. To advance GA research and enhance patient outcomes, cooperation between funding agencies, researchers, and advocacy groups is important.

Clinical Trials and Ethical Issues

Informed permission from patients, safety monitoring, data integrity, and openness in outcome reporting are all ethical factors to be taken into account in GA clinical studies. To protect patient safety and study integrity, researchers follow legal requirements and ethical principles. To produce findings that may be applied broadly, clinical trial inclusion criteria are created to strike a compromise between patient diversity and scientific rigor.

Opportunities for Translational Research

Clinical applications in GA management are connected to basic science discoveries through translational research. This involves moving tailored medicines from the bench to the bedside, creating biomarker-driven diagnostic tools, and verifying preclinical findings in human investigations. Collaborations in translational research expedite the conversion of scientific information into concrete advantages for patients with GA.

Prospects for Granuloma Annulare Management in the Future

Approaches to granuloma annulare management in the future should be tailored, focused, and comprehensive. This involves applying precision medicine techniques for medication selection, incorporating patient-centered care models, and utilizing biomarkers for early diagnosis and prognostication. Technological developments in patient education, telemedicine, and digital health empower patients and improve GA healthcare delivery.

The combined goal of these research developments and future paths is to revolutionize the management of granuloma annulare, promoting creativity, enhancing results, and eventually helping patients and healthcare communities across the globe.

www.ingramcontent.com/pod-product-compliance
Lightning Source LLC
Chambersburg PA
CBHW071834210526
45479CB00001B/130